Migraine

All you need to know

Dr. Sheila Harrison

Disclaimer

This content serves to provide general information about the disease and aims to empower you to seek prompt medical assistance if necessary to prevent complications. It's essential to stress that this information is not a substitute for consulting a qualified physician. The field of medical science is continually evolving, and due to the dynamic nature of medical knowledge, we recommend seeking expert advice if you encounter any inconsistencies or intend to take action based on the information in this content. Never disregard professional medical guidance or delay treatment based on something you've read online, including this material, or from any other online source. Always remember that the internet cannot cure you; rather, healing comes through the guidance of medical professionals and the providence of God.

Table of contents

Overview

A migraine is much more than a bad headache. This neurological disease can cause debilitating throbbing pain that can leave you in bed for days! Movement, light, sound and other triggers may cause symptoms like pain, tiredness, nausea, visual disturbances, numbness and tingling, irritability, difficulty speaking, temporary loss of vision and many more.

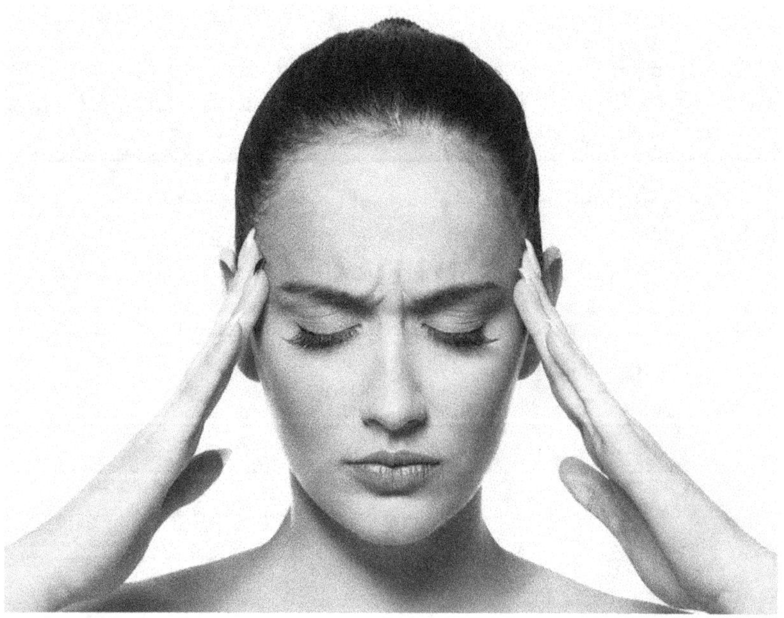

How often do migraines happen?

The frequency of a migraine could be once a year, once a week or any amount of time in between. Having two to four migraine headaches per month is the most common.

Can children get migraines?

Yes, but pediatric migraines are often shorter and there are more stomach symptoms.

Who should I see about my migraine pain?

Discuss your symptoms with your primary care provider first. They can diagnose migraine headaches and start treatment. You may require a referral to a headache specialist.

Do migraines cause permanent brain damage?

No. Migraines don't cause brain damage.

There is a tiny risk of stroke in people who get migraines with aura – 1 or 2 people out of 100,000.

Section 1

What is Migraine ?

A migraine is a common neurological disease that causes a variety of symptoms, most notably a throbbing, pulsing headache on one side of your head. Your migraine will likely get worse with physical activity, lights, sounds or smells. It may last at least four hours or even days. About 12% of Americans have this genetic disorder. Research shows that it's the sixth most disabling disease in the world.

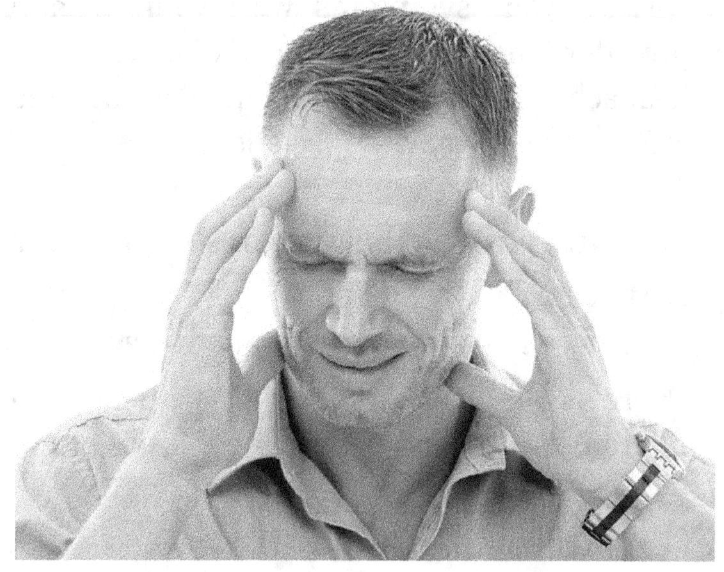

Migraine is a complex disorder characterized by recurrent episodes of headache, most often unilateral and in some cases associated with visual or sensory symptoms—collectively known as an aura—that arise most often before the head pain but that may occur during or afterward (see the image below). Migraine is most common in women and has a strong genetic component.

Migraine is a kind of strong throbbing or pulsating headache on one side of the head. It is usually accompanied by nausea, vomiting and an increase in light and sound sensitivity. Migraine attacks can last anywhere from hours to days, and the pain may be severe enough to prevent you from going about your usual activities.

A migraine can be associated with a symptom known as an aura that might appear before or with a headache in some people. Visual problems, such as flashes of light or blind spots, or other problems, such as tingling on one side of the face, arm, or leg, and difficulty speaking, can all occur during a migraine.

Migraine is a special kind of headache. Severe cases can have a negative impact on a person's day-to-day life, hindering their ability to work or study.

It affects different people differently, with variable triggers, severity, symptoms, and frequency. Some people have many episodes per week, while others have them occasionally. Medications can help prevent and alleviate the pain of some migraines. The best treatment is usually a combination of medications with lifestyle adjustments.

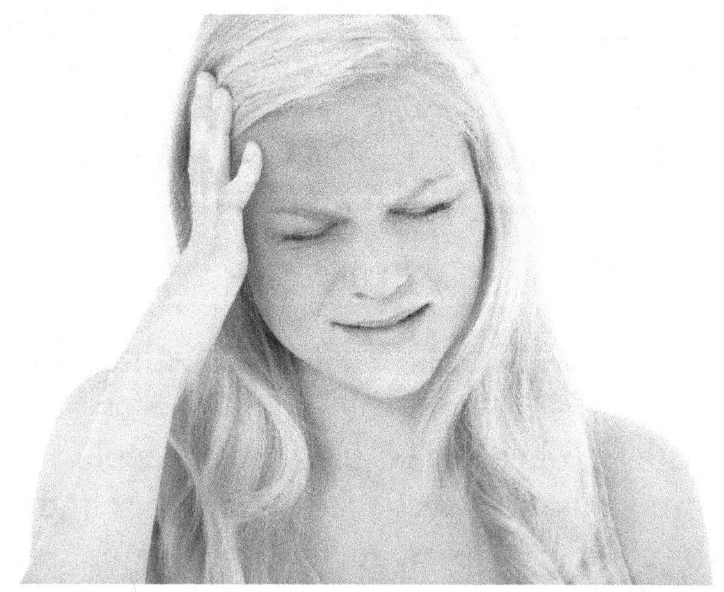

An aura

An aura is a group of sensory, motor and speech symptoms that usually act like warning signals that a migraine headache is about to begin. Commonly misinterpreted as a seizure or stroke, it typically happens before the headache pain, but can sometimes appear during or even after. An aura can last from 10 to 60 minutes. About 15% to 20% of people who experience migraines have auras.

Aura symptoms are reversible, meaning that they can be stopped/healed. An aura produces symptoms that may include:

- Seeing bright flashing dots, sparkles, or lights.
- Blind spots in your vision.
- Numb or tingling skin.
- Speech changes.
- Ringing in your ears (tinnitus).
- Temporary vision loss.
- Seeing wavy or jagged lines.
- Changes in smell or taste.
- A "funny" feeling.

Section 2

Types of Migraines

There are several types of migraines, and the same type may go by different names:

- **Migraine with aura (complicated migraine):** Around 15% to 20% of people with migraine headaches experience an aura.

- **Migraine without aura (common migraine):** This type of migraine headache strikes without the warning an aura may give you. The symptoms are the same, but that phase doesn't happen.

- **Migraine without head pain:** "Silent migraine" or "acephalgic migraine," as this type is also known as, includes the aura symptom but not the headache that typically follows.

- **Hemiplegic migraine:** You'll have temporary paralysis (hemiplegia) or neurological or sensory changes on one side of your body.

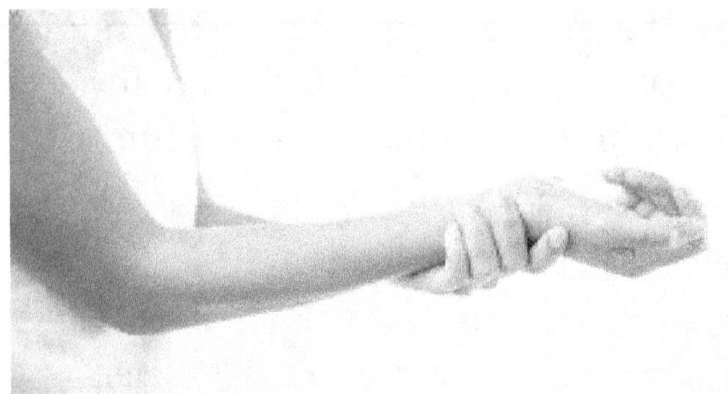

The onset of the headache may be associated with temporary numbness, extreme weakness on one side of your body, a tingling sensation, a loss of sensation and dizziness or vision changes. Sometimes it includes head pain and sometimes it doesn't.

- **Retinal migraine (ocular migraine):** You may notice temporary, partial or complete loss of vision in one of your eyes, along with a dull ache behind the eye that may spread to the rest of your head.

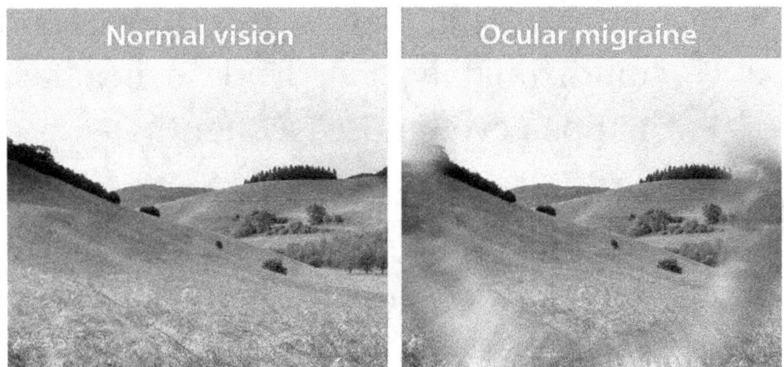

That vision loss may last a minute, or as long as months. You should always report a retinal migraine to a healthcare provider because it could be a sign of a more serious issue.

- **Chronic migraine:** A chronic migraine is when a migraine occurs at least 15 days per month. The symptoms may change frequently, and so may the severity of the pain.

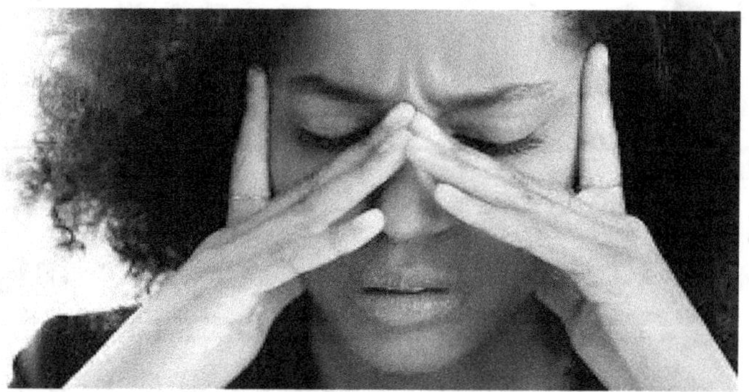

Those who get chronic migraines might be using headache pain medications more than 10 to 15 days a month and that, unfortunately, can lead to headaches that happen even more frequently.

- **Migraine with brainstem aura:** With this migraine, you'll have vertigo, slurred speech, double vision or loss of balance, which occur before the headache. The headache pain may affect the back of your head.

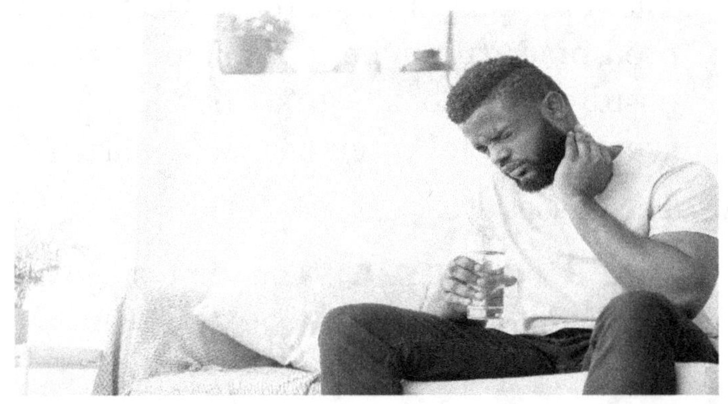

These symptoms usually occur suddenly and can be associated with the inability to speak properly, ringing in the ears and vomiting.

- **Status migrainosus:** This is a rare and severe type of migraine that can last longer than 72 hours. The headache pain and nausea can be extremely bad. Certain medications, or medication withdrawal, can cause you to have this type of migraine.

The four stages or phases of a migraine their timeline

The four stages in chronological order are the prodrome (pre-monitory), aura, headache and postdrome. About 30% of people experience symptoms before their headache starts.

The phases are:

1. **Prodrome:** The first stage lasts a few hours, or it can last days.

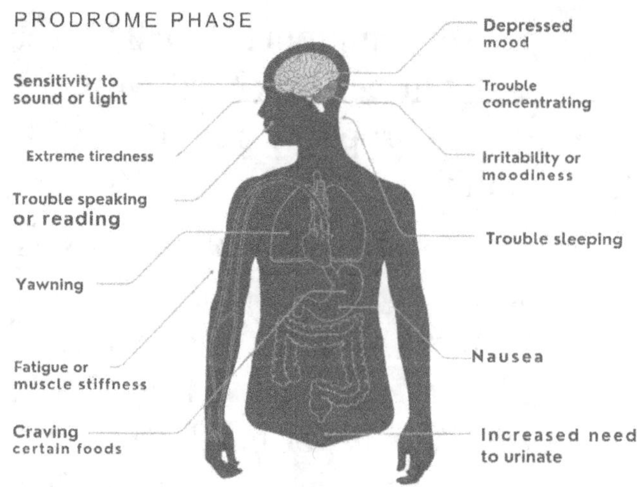

   You may or may not experience it as it may not happen every time. Some know it as the "pre headache" or "premonitory" phase.

2. **Aura:** The aura phase can last as long as 60 minutes or as little as five.

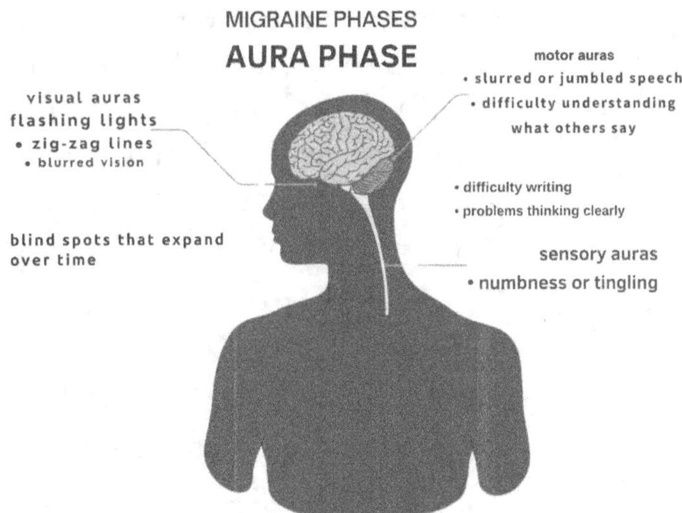

Most people don't experience an aura, and some have both the aura and the headache at the same time.

3. **Headache:** About four hours to 72 hours is how long the headache lasts.

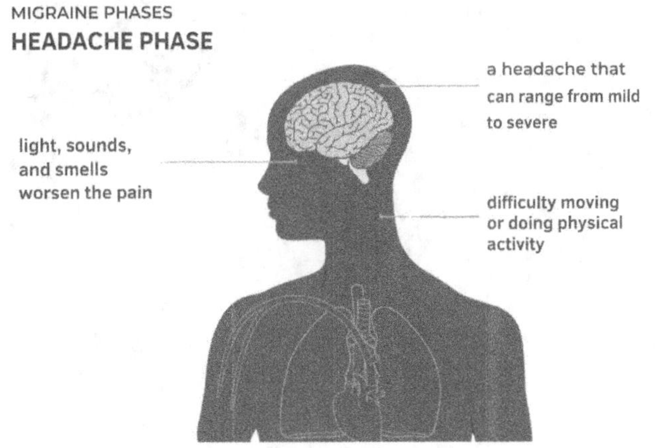

The word "ache" doesn't do the pain justice because sometimes it's mild, but usually, it's described as drilling, throbbing or you may feel the sensation of an icepick in your head. Typically it starts on one side of your head and then spreads to the other side.

4. **Postdrome:** The postdrome stage goes on for a day or two. It's often called a migraine "hangover" and 80% of those who have migraines experience it.

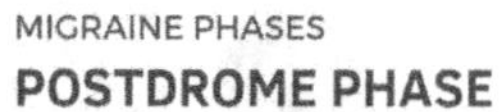

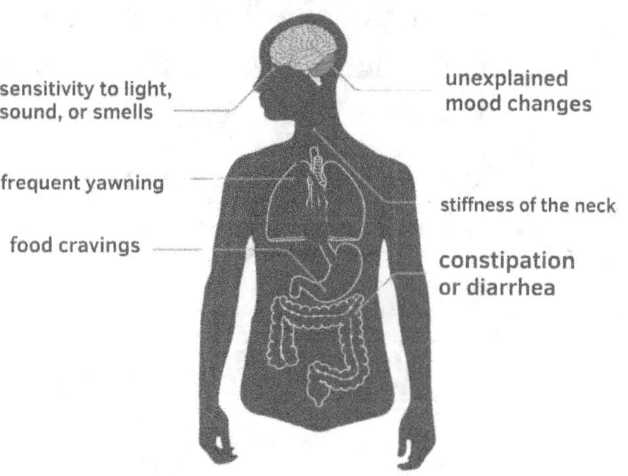

Section 3

Signs / Symptoms of Migraine

The primary symptom of migraine is a headache. Pain is sometimes described as pounding or throbbing. It can begin as a dull ache that develops into pulsing pain that is mild, moderate or severe. If left untreated, your headache pain will become moderate to severe. Pain can shift from one side of your head to the other, or it can affect the front of your head, the back of your head or feel like it's affecting your whole head. Some people feel pain around their eye or temple, and sometimes in their face, sinuses, jaw or neck.

Other symptoms of migraine headaches include:

- Sensitivity to light, noise and odors.

- Nausea and vomiting, upset stomach and abdominal pain. Nausea (80%) and vomiting (50%), including anorexia and food intolerance, and light-headedness

- Unilateral and localized pain in the frontotemporal and ocular area, but the pain may be felt anywhere around the head or neck.

- Headache lasts 4–72 hours

- Pain builds up over a period of 1–2 hours, progressing posteriorly and becoming diffuse
- Loss of appetite.
- Feeling very warm (sweating) or cold (chills).
- Pale skin color (pallor).
- Feeling tired.
- Dizziness and blurred vision.
- Tender scalp.
- Diarrhea (rare).
- Fever (rare).

Most migraines last about four hours, although severe ones can last much longer.

Each phase of the migraine attack can come with different symptoms:

Prodrome symptoms:

- Problems concentrating.
- Irritability and/or depression.
- Difficulty speaking and reading.
- Difficulty sleeping. Yawning.
- Nausea.
- Fatigue.
- Sensitivity to light and sound.
- Food cravings.

- Increased urination.
- Muscle stiffness.

Aura symptoms:

- May precede or accompany the headache phase or may occur in isolation.
- Usually develops over 5–20 minutes and lasts less than 60 minutes
- Numbness and tingling.
- Visual disturbances. You might be seeing the world as if through a kaleidoscope, have blurry spots or see sparkles or lines. Visual symptoms may be positive or negative
- Temporary loss of sight. The most common positive visual phenomenon is the scintillating scotoma, an arc or band of absent vision with a shimmering or glittering zigzag border
- Weakness on one side of the body.
- Speech changes.

Headache symptoms:

- Neck pain, stiffness.
- Depression, giddiness and/or anxiety.
- Sensitivity to light, smell and sound.

- ■ Nasal congestion.
- ■ Insomnia.
- ■ Nausea and vomiting.

Postdrome symptoms:

- ■ Inability to concentrate.
- ■ Depressed mood.
- ■ Fatigue.
- ■ Lack of comprehension.
- ■ Euphoric mood.

Physical findings during a migraine headache may include the following:

- Cranial/cervical muscle tenderness
- Horner syndrome (ie, relative miosis with 1–2 mm of ptosis on the same side as the headache)
- Conjunctival injection
- Tachycardia or bradycardia
- Hypertension or hypotension
- Hemisensory or hemiparetic neurologic deficits (ie, complicated migraine)
- Adie-type pupil (ie, poor light reactivity, with near dissociation from light)

Section 4

Migraine Triggers

Migraine attacks can be triggered by a variety of factors. Common triggers include:

- **Emotional stress:** Emotional stress is one of the most common triggers of migraine headaches. During stressful events, certain chemicals in the brain are released to combat the situation (known as the "flight or fight" response). The release of these chemicals can bring on a migraine. Other emotions like anxiety, worry and excitement can increase muscle tension and dilate blood vessels. That can make your migraine more severe.
- **Missing a meal:** Delaying a meal might also trigger your migraine headache.
- **Sensitivity to specific chemicals and preservatives in foods:** Certain foods and beverages such as aged cheese, beverages containing alcohol, chocolate and food additives such as nitrates (found in pepperoni, hot dogs and luncheon meats) and fermented or pickled foods may

be responsible for triggering up to 30% of migraines.

- **Caffeine:** Having too much caffeine or withdrawal from caffeine can cause headaches when the caffeine level abruptly drops. Your blood vessels seem to become sensitized to caffeine and when you don't get it, a headache may occur. Caffeine is sometimes recommended by healthcare providers to help with treating acute migraine attacks but should not be used frequently.

- **Alcohol:** Alcohol, particularly wine can also trigger migraine.

- **Sleep patterns shift**: Sleep deprivation or more sleep can cause migraines in certain people.

- **Daily use of pain-relieving medications:** If you use medicine meant to relieve headache pain too often, that can cause a rebound headache.

- **Certain Medical Conditions:** Migraines can be associated with some medical conditions, such as sleep disorders, high blood pressure, and anxiety.

- **Hormonal changes in women:** Migraines in women are more common around the time of their menstrual periods. The abrupt drop in estrogen that triggers menses can also trigger migraines. Hormonal changes can also be brought on by birth control pills and hormone replacement therapy. Migraines are generally worse between puberty and menopause since these estrogen fluctuations generally don't occur in young girls and post-menopausal women. If your hormones are a strong factor in your migraines, you may have fewer headaches after menopause. Hormonal changes do not appear to trigger migraines in men.
- **Light:** Flashing lights, fluorescent lights, light from the TV or computer and sunlight can trigger you.

Other possible triggers include:

- Changing weather conditions such as storm fronts, barometric pressure changes, strong winds or changes in altitude.

- Being overly tired. Overexertion.
- Dieting, or not drinking enough water.
- Loud noises.
- Exposure to smoke, perfumes or other odors.
- Certain medications cause blood vessels to swell.
- Pollen, dust, and other allergens can act as triggers.
- Medication side effects: Certain medications, such as vasodilators and oral contraceptives, can trigger migraines.

Section 5

Causes of Migraine

While the exact etiology of migraines is unknown, genetic and environmental factors appear to play a role.

Genetic Predisposition

Family history can play a significant role, as individuals with a family history of migraines are more likely to experience them.

Neurological Factors

1. Abnormal brain activity: Migraines may result from changes in brain activity affecting blood flow and nerve signaling.

2. Imbalance in brain chemicals: Serotonin, a neurotransmitter, appears to be involved in migraine development. Changes in its levels can trigger an attack.

3. The trigeminal nerve which carries sensory messages from the face and helps in the functioning of the jaw has been implicated in migraine.

4. Other neurotransmitters, such as calcitonin gene-related peptides also play a role in migraines (CGRP).

Hormonal Changes

1. Hormonal fluctuations: Migraines are more common in women, often related to hormonal changes during the menstrual cycle, pregnancy, or menopause.

2. Hormone therapy and birth control: Some hormone-based medications can trigger migraines in susceptible individuals.

Environmental Triggers

1. Certain foods and drinks: Common dietary triggers include alcohol (especially red wine), caffeine, aged cheeses, processed foods, and artificial sweeteners.

2. Skipping meals: Low blood sugar from missed meals can trigger migraines.

3. Dehydration: Inadequate fluid intake can lead to migraines.

4. Strong odors and chemicals: Perfumes, strong-smelling cleaning products, and exposure to certain chemicals can be triggers.

5. Weather changes: Sudden weather changes, high humidity, or changes in barometric pressure can provoke migraines.

Sensory Stimuli

1. Bright lights and glare: Exposure to bright lights, flickering screens, or direct sunlight can trigger migraines.
2. Loud noises: Noise from music, construction work, or other sources can be a trigger.

Physical Factors

1. Lack of sleep or irregular sleep patterns can increase the risk of migraines.
2. Overexertion or physical strain, including intense exercise, can trigger an attack.
3. Physical or emotional stress can be a major factor in migraine onset.

Section 6

Risk Factors for Migraine

Migraines can affect people of all ages, genders, and backgrounds. While anyone can experience a migraine, certain risk factors and predisposing conditions can make some individuals more susceptible to developing migraines. Here are some common risk factors associated with migraines:

- **Family History:** A family history of migraines can significantly increase an individual's risk of developing them. Genetic factors may play a role in migraine susceptibility.

- **Gender:** Migraines are more prevalent in women than in men. This gender difference may be related to hormonal fluctuations, as migraines are often associated with the menstrual cycle.

- **Hormonal Changes:** Hormonal fluctuations can trigger migraines in some individuals. For women, this includes menstruation, pregnancy, menopause, and the use of oral contraceptives or hormone replacement therapy.

- **Age:** Migraines can start at any age, but they often develop during adolescence or early adulthood. Some individuals may experience their first migraine later in life.

- **Other Medical Conditions:** Certain medical conditions and comorbidities can increase the risk of migraines, including:
  - Anxiety and depression
  - Sleep disorders, such as insomnia or sleep apnea
  - High blood pressure
  - Stroke or cardiovascular diseases
  - Epilepsy

- **Medication Overuse:** Overusing pain-relief medications, including those used to treat migraines, can lead to medication-overuse headaches and increase the frequency and severity of migraines.

- **Obesity:** Studies have shown a potential link between obesity and an increased risk of migraines. Managing weight through a healthy lifestyle may help reduce migraine frequency.

- **Smoking and Alcohol:** Both smoking and excessive alcohol consumption are associated with a higher risk of migraines. These lifestyle factors can trigger or worsen migraine attacks.

- **Dietary Factors:** Certain foods and food additives are known migraine triggers for some individuals. Common dietary triggers include alcohol, caffeine, aged cheeses, processed foods, and artificial sweeteners.

- **Environmental Factors:** Sensitivity to environmental factors such as strong odors, bright lights, and loud noises can contribute to migraines.

- **Stress:** High levels of stress and emotional tension are common migraine triggers. Stress management techniques may help reduce the risk.

- **Physical Exertion:** Strenuous physical activity, especially if not accustomed to it, can trigger exercise-induced migraines in some individuals.

It's important to note that while these risk factors can increase an individual's likelihood of experiencing migraines, many people with migraines do not have any specific risk factors. Migraines are a complex neurological condition with various contributing factors, and their triggers and patterns can vary widely from person to person.

Section 7

Complications Associated with Migraine

Migraines are more than just severe headaches; they can be accompanied by various complications and related symptoms that significantly impact a person's life. Here are some of the complications and associated issues that can arise with migraines:

- **Chronic Migraines:** Some individuals experience chronic migraines, characterized by headaches on 15 or more days per month for at least three months. This condition can lead to a reduced quality of life and increased disability.

- **Medication Overuse Headache (MOH):** Overusing pain relief medications for migraines can paradoxically lead to more frequent or severe headaches. This condition is known as MOH or rebound headache.

- **Stroke:** Patients with migraine have a small chance of developing a stroke

- **Epilepsy:** An episode of migraine may rarely result in a seizure

- Some episodes of migraine do not respond to treatment and can persist without relief for very long durations.

- **Status Migrainosus:** A status migrainosus is a rare and severe type of migraine that lasts longer than 72 hours and does not respond well to treatment. It can lead to dehydration, severe pain, and hospitalization.

- **Secondary Complications:** Migraine attacks may lead to secondary complications, including dehydration from vomiting, fatigue, and irritability due to disrupted sleep patterns, and difficulty focusing or concentrating.

- **Safety Concerns:** Visual disturbances or cognitive impairments during migraine attacks can pose safety risks, especially if a person is driving or operating heavy machinery.

- **Increased Risk of Other Health Issues:** Research suggests that individuals with migraines may have a higher risk of developing other health issues, such as cardiovascular diseases or mental health conditions.

Section 8

Diagnosis for Migraine

Diagnosing migraines involves a thorough evaluation by a healthcare professional to rule out other possible causes of headache and to determine if the symptoms fit the criteria for migraines. And so migraine is a clinical diagnosis that a doctor will make based on your symptoms. However, imaging may be performed on those who do not respond to treatment to look for other causes of headaches.

- **Medical History:** The healthcare provider will begin by taking a detailed medical history, including the patient's personal and family medical history, as migraines can have a genetic component.

- **Symptom Description**: The patient will be asked to describe their headache symptoms in detail, including the frequency, duration, location, type of pain, and any associated symptoms such as aura, nausea, vomiting, or sensitivity to light and sound. To diagnose a migraine, your healthcare provider will get a thorough medical history, not just your history of headaches but your family's, too. Also, they'll want to establish a history of your migraine-related symptoms, likely asking you to:

- Describe your headache symptoms. How severe are they?
- Remember when you get them. During your period, for example?
- Describe the type and location of your pain. Is the pain pounding? Pulsing? Throbbing?
- Remember if anything makes your headache better or worse.
- Tell how often you get migraine headaches.
- Talk about the activities, foods, stressors or the situations that may have brought on the migraine.
- Discuss what medications you take to relieve the pain and how often you take them.
- Tell how you felt before, during and after the headache.
- Remember if anyone in your family gets migraine headaches.

■ **Physical Examination:** A physical examination will be conducted to check for any neurological abnormalities and to rule out other underlying health conditions.

- **Differential Diagnosis:** The healthcare provider will consider other possible causes of headaches and rule them out. This may involve tests to exclude conditions like tension-type headaches, cluster headaches, or other neurological disorders.

- **Blood Tests:** Blood tests may be conducted to check for any underlying conditions or to rule out other medical issues.

- **Magnetic resonance imaging (MRI):** MRI scan creates comprehensive images of the brain and its arteries using a high magnetic field and radio waves.

- **CT scan (computerized tomography):** CT scan induces comprehensive cross-sectional images of the brain using a succession of X-rays.

- **Migraine Specialist Consultation:** In cases where the diagnosis is challenging or there is a need for specialized care, a consultation with a headache specialist or neurologist who specializes in migraine management may be recommended.

Migraine Journal

- Keeping a migraine journal is not only beneficial to you, but it helps your healthcare provider with the diagnosis process. Your journal should be detailed and updated as much as possible before, during and after a migraine attack. Consider keeping track of the following:

- The date and time of when the migraine began – specifically when the prodrome started, if you're able to tell it's happening. Track time passing. When did the aura phase begin? The headache? The postdrome? Do your best to tell what stage you're in and how long it lasts. If there's a pattern, that may help you anticipate what will happen in the future.

- What are your symptoms? Be specific.

- Note how many hours of sleep you got the night before it happened and your stress level. What's causing your stress?

- Note the weather.

- Log your food and water intake. Did you eat something that triggered the migraine? Did you miss a meal?

- Describe the type of pain and rate it on a one to 10 scale with 10 being the worst pain you've ever experienced.

- Where is the pain located? One side of your head? Your jaw? Your eyes?

- List all of the medications you took. This includes any daily prescriptions, any supplements and any pain medication you took.

- How did you try to treat your migraine, and did it work? What medicine did you take, at what dosage, at what time?

- Consider other triggers. Maybe you played basketball in the sunlight? Maybe you watched a movie that had flashing lights? If you're a woman, are you on your period?

There are some smartphone apps you can use to keep a migraine journal if you don't want to use pen and paper.

Section 9

Treatment of Migraine

The goal of migraine treatment is to alleviate symptoms and avoid future attacks. There are two kinds of migraine medications:

- **Analgesics (pain relievers):** These medications, often a part of acute or abortive treatment, are administered during migraine attacks and are intended to relieve symptoms.

- **Medication for prevention:** To minimize the severity or frequency of migraines, these medications are used on a regular basis, often daily.

The frequency and severity of headaches, coupled with whether or not they are accompanied by nausea and vomiting, the degree of disability they cause and any other medical issues experienced are all factors that influence treatment options.

Medications for Migraine Relief

Over-the-counter medications are effective for some people with mild to moderate migraines. The main ingredients in pain relieving medications are ibuprofen, aspirin, acetaminophen, naproxen and caffeine.

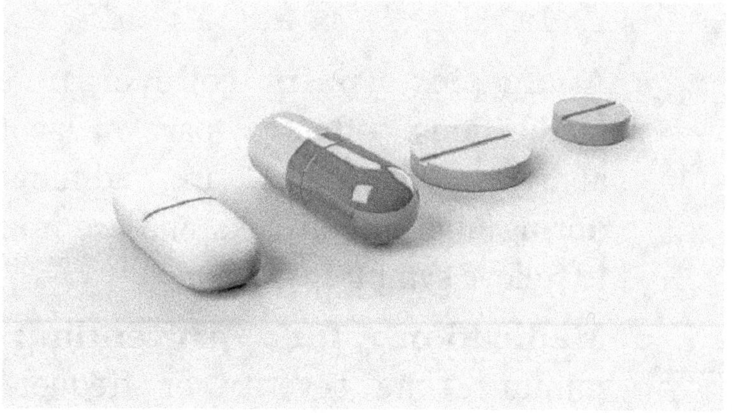

Three over-the-counter products approved by the Food and Drug Administration for migraine headaches are:

- Excedrin® Migraine.
- Advil® Migraine.
- Motrin® Migraine Pain.

Be cautious when taking over-the-counter pain relieving medications. Sometimes overusing them can cause analgesic-rebound headaches or a dependency problem. If you're taking any over-the-counter pain medications more than two to three times a week, report that to your healthcare provider. They may suggest prescription medications that may be more effective.

Prescription drugs for migraine headaches include:

Triptan class of drugs (these are abortives):
- Sumatriptan.
- Zolmitriptan.
- Naratriptan.

Calcium channel blockers:
- Verapamil.

Calcitonin gene-related (CGRP) monoclonal antibodies:
- Erenumab.
- Fremanezumab.
- Galcanezumab.
- Eptinezumab.

Beta blockers:
- Atenolol.
- Propranolol.
- Nadolol.

Antidepressants:

- Amitriptyline.
- Nortriptyline.
- Doxepin.
- Venlafaxine.
- Duloxetine.

Antiseizure drugs:

- Valproic acid.
- Topiramate.

Other:

- Steroids.
- Phenothiazines.
- Corticosteroids.

Your healthcare provider might recommend vitamins, minerals, or herbs, including:

- Riboflavin (vitamin B2).
- Magnesium.
- Feverfew.
- Butterbur.
- Co-enzyme Q10.

Drugs to relieve migraine pain come in a variety of formulations including pills, tablets, injections, suppositories and nasal sprays. You and your healthcare provider will discuss the specific medication, combination of medications and formulations to best meet your unique headache pain. Drugs to relieve nausea are also prescribed, if needed.

All medications should be used under the direction of a headache specialist or healthcare provider familiar with migraine therapy. As with any medication, it's important to carefully follow the label instructions and your healthcare provider's advice.

Alternative migraine management methods, also known as home remedies, include:

- Resting in a dark, quiet, cool room.
- Applying a cold compress or washcloth to your forehead or behind your neck. (Some people prefer heat.)
- Massaging your scalp.
- Yoga.
- Applying pressure to your temples in a circular motion.
- Keep yourself in a calm state. Meditating.
- Biofeedback.

Section 10
Prevention of Migraine

- **Sleep:** Every day, including weekends and holidays, go to bed and wake up at the same hour.

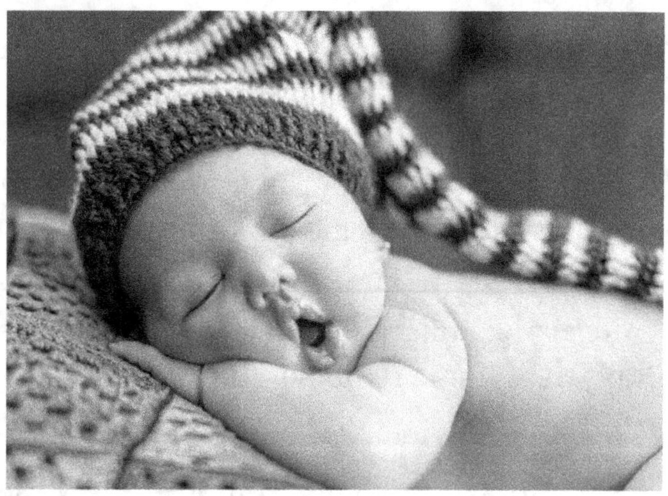

  A headache might be triggered when you fall asleep at unusual times or when you receive too much or too little sleep. Get seven to nine hours of sleep a night.

- **Exercise on a regular basis:** You may be tempted to avoid physical activity for fear of triggering a migraine.

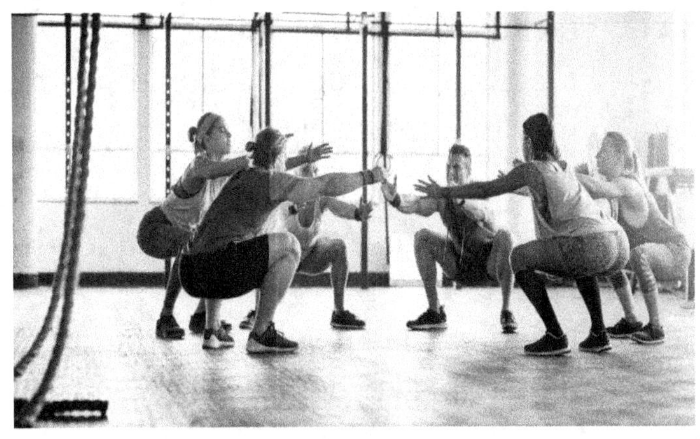

For some people, overdoing a workout might cause a headache, but evidence shows that regular, moderate aerobic activity can help migraine episodes be shorter, less painful, and less frequent. It also aids in the management of stress, which can be a trigger.

- **Eat at regular intervals:** A migraine might be triggered by a dip in blood sugar, so do not miss meals. Drink plenty of water to avoid dehydration, which can also set off an episode.

- **Keep stress to a minimum:** Stress is a typical cause of anxiety. Allowing some time each day to unwind may help alleviate stress and manage anxiety. Learn techniques to control stress such as meditation, yoga, relaxation training, or mindful breathing.

- Reduction of migraine triggers (eg, lack of sleep, fatigue, stress, certain foods)

- Nonpharmacologic therapy (eg, biofeedback, cognitive-behavioral therapy)

- Integrative medicine (eg, butterbur, riboflavin, magnesium, feverfew, coenzyme Q10)

- Keep a migraine diary. Take notes about any foods and other triggers that you think may have caused you to develop a migraine. Make changes in your diet and avoid those triggers as much as possible.
- Get a prescription for CGRP monoclonal antibodies. This injection was created specifically to help with migraines.
- Take medications as directed by your healthcare provider. Preventative medications include antidepressants, anti-seizure medications, calcitonin gene-related peptides, medicines that lower blood pressure and Botox injections. You

might be prescribed timolol, amitriptyline, topiramate and divalproex sodium. Notice that some of the same medications that can help you manage a migraine may also help prevent one.

- Talk to your healthcare provider about hormone therapy if your migraines are thought to be linked to your menstrual cycle.
- Consider trying a transcutaneous supraorbital nerve stimulation device. This battery-powered electrical stimulator device is approved by the Food and Drug Administration to prevent migraines. The device, worn like a headband or on your arm, emits electrical charges. The charge stimulates the nerve that transmits some of the pain experienced in migraine headaches. (The device may not be covered by your health insurance.)
- Get counseling from a therapist for help controlling your stress. Ask your healthcare provider for a referral.

www.ingramcontent.com/pod-product-compliance
Lightning Source LLC
Chambersburg PA
CBHW070741260726
48660CB00007B/2924